Staying Healthy

Together We Can: Pandemic

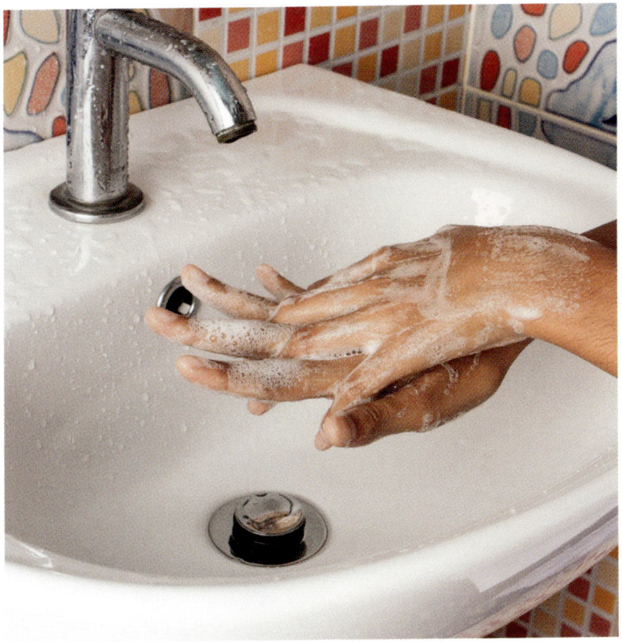

By Shannon Stocker

21st Century Junior Library

CHERRY LAKE PRESS

Published in the United States of America by Cherry Lake Publishing Group
Ann Arbor, Michigan
www.cherrylakepublishing.com

Reading Adviser: Marla Conn, MS, Ed., Literacy specialist, Read-Ability, Inc.

Photo Credits: © Pikul Noorod/Shutterstock.com, cover, 1; © Charles Lewis/Shutterstock.com, 4; © Shampanskiy/Shutterstock.com, 6; © Viktar Malyshchyts/Shutterstock.com, 8; © AP_FOOTAGE/Shutterstock.com, 10; © Volurol/Shutterstock.com, 12; © Kits Pix/Shutterstock.com, 14; © KlingSup/Shutterstock.com, 16; © Monkey Business Images/Shutterstock.com, 18; © Monkey Business Images/Shutterstock.com, 20

Cherry Lake Press is an imprint of Cherry Lake Publishing Group.

Library of Congress Cataloging-in-Publication Data

Names: Stocker, Shannon, author.
Title: Staying healthy / Shannon Stocker.
Description: Ann Arbor, Michigan : Cherry Lake Publishing, 2021. | Series: Together we can: pandemic | Includes index. | Audience: Grades 2-3 | Summary: "The COVID-19 pandemic introduced many changes into children's lives. Staying Healthy give readers the tools they need to reduce risk for themselves and their families. Actionable suggestions help young readers adapt and cope as we navigate the current outbreak. This book includes science content, based on current CDC recommendations, as well as social emotional content to help with personal wellness and development of empathy. All books in the 21st Century Junior Library encourage readers to think critically and creatively, and use their problem-solving skills. Book includes table of contents, sidebars, glossary, index, and author biography"—Provided by publisher.
Identifiers: LCCN 2020039983 (print) | LCCN 2020039984 (ebook) | ISBN 9781534180130 (hardcover) | ISBN 9781534181847 (paperback) | ISBN 9781534181144 (pdf) | ISBN 9781534182851 (ebook)
Subjects: LCSH: Health—Juvenile literature. | Hygiene—Juvenile literature.
Classification: LCC RA777 .S817 2021 (print) | LCC RA777 (ebook) | DDC 613—dc23
LC record available at https://lccn.loc.gov/2020039983
LC ebook record available at https://lccn.loc.gov/2020039984

Cherry Lake Publishing Group would like to acknowledge the work of the Partnership for 21st Century Learning, a Network of Battelle for Kids. Please visit http://www.battelleforkids.org/networks/p21 for more information.

Printed in the United States of America
Corporate Graphics

CONTENTS

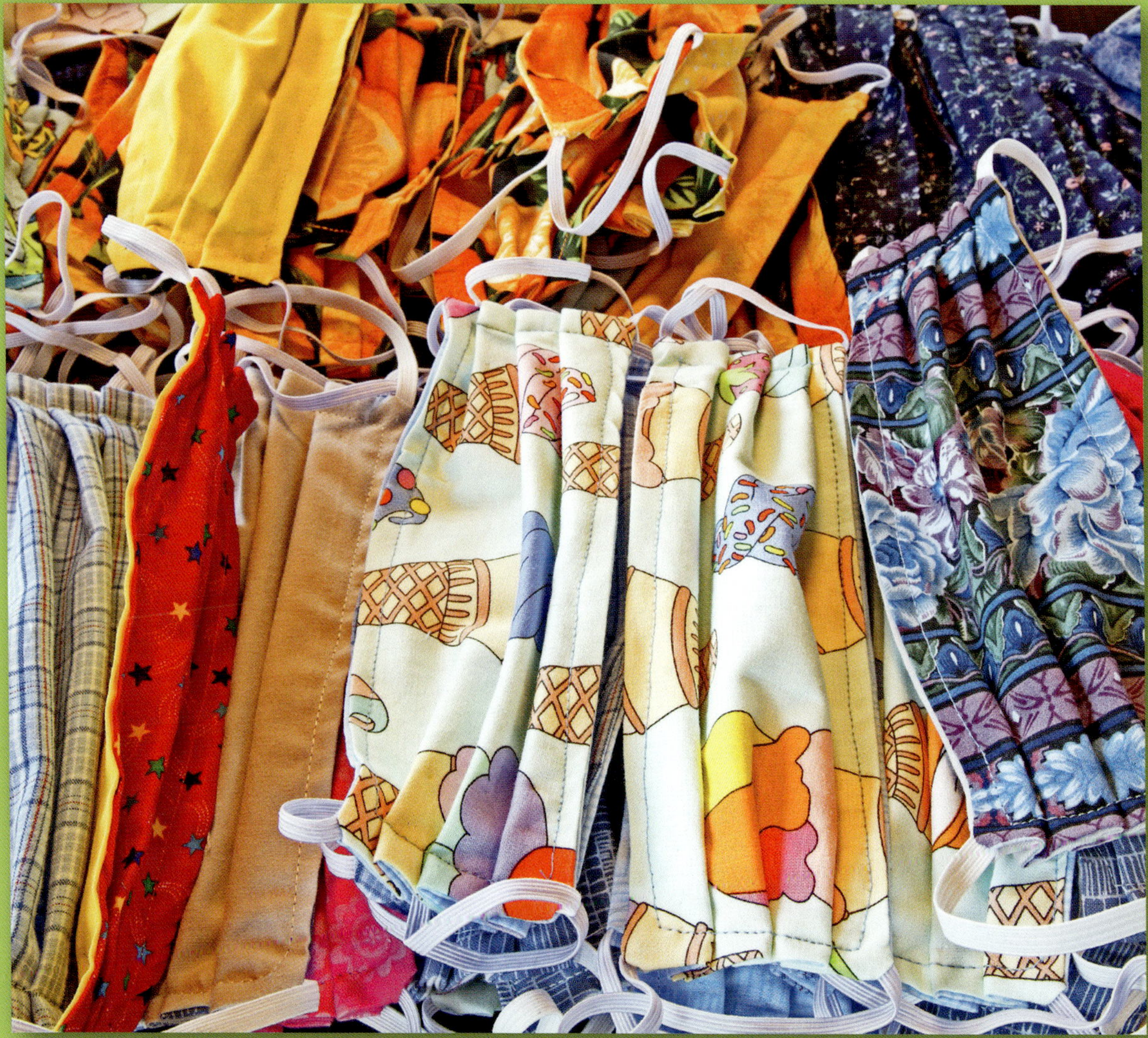

Cloth masks are both comfortable and washable.

Healthy at Home

Staying healthy during a **pandemic**, like the **coronavirus**, can mean different things to different people. For example, some people will wear masks while others will not. Some friends have playdates at home while others practice **social distancing**. It can all be confusing. So what *should* we be doing to best protect ourselves and others?

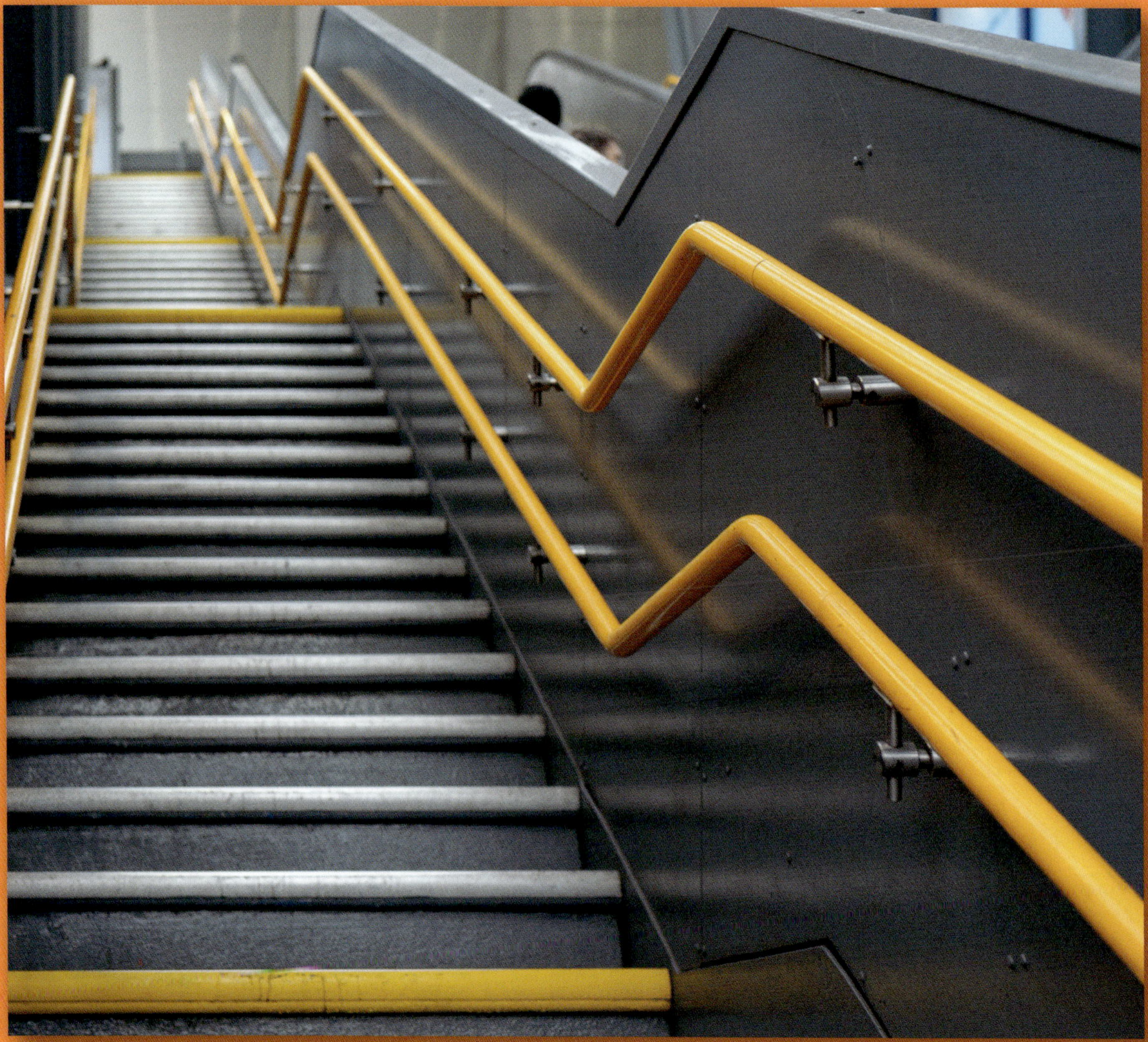

When out in public, try not to touch common surfaces like railings and doorknobs.

Staying healthy at home should always start with good **hygiene**. Examples of good hygiene are taking regular baths, wearing clean clothes, and washing your hands frequently. Wash your hands with soap and water for at least 20 seconds, and make sure you clean under your nails with a brush or washcloth. Don't forget to wash your thumbs too!

Sing!

Did you know that it takes about 20 seconds to sing your ABCs?

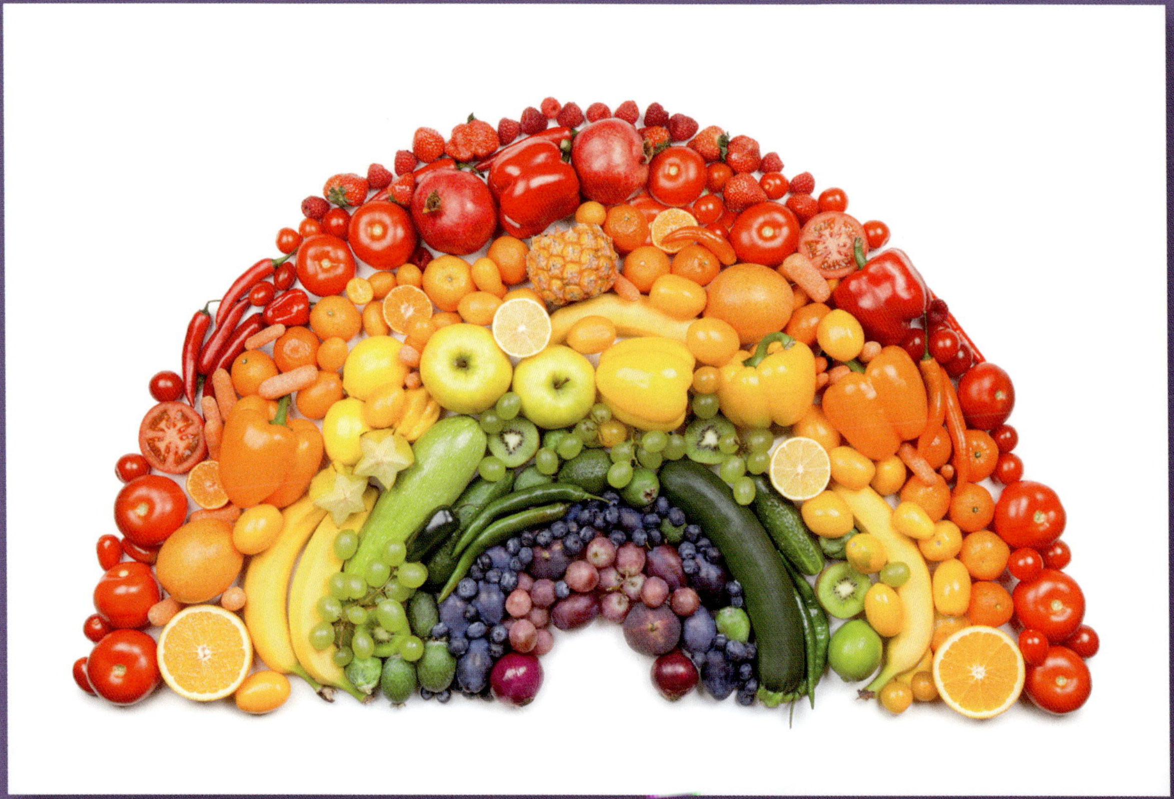

Try eating a rainbow of fruits and vegetables!

Just because you're **quarantined** doesn't mean you shouldn't eat healthy foods and exercise! Staying healthy at home means taking care of the inside of your body too. Healthy meals and snacks should include vegetables, fruits, whole grains, and proteins whenever possible. And don't forget to do some kind of exercise every day!

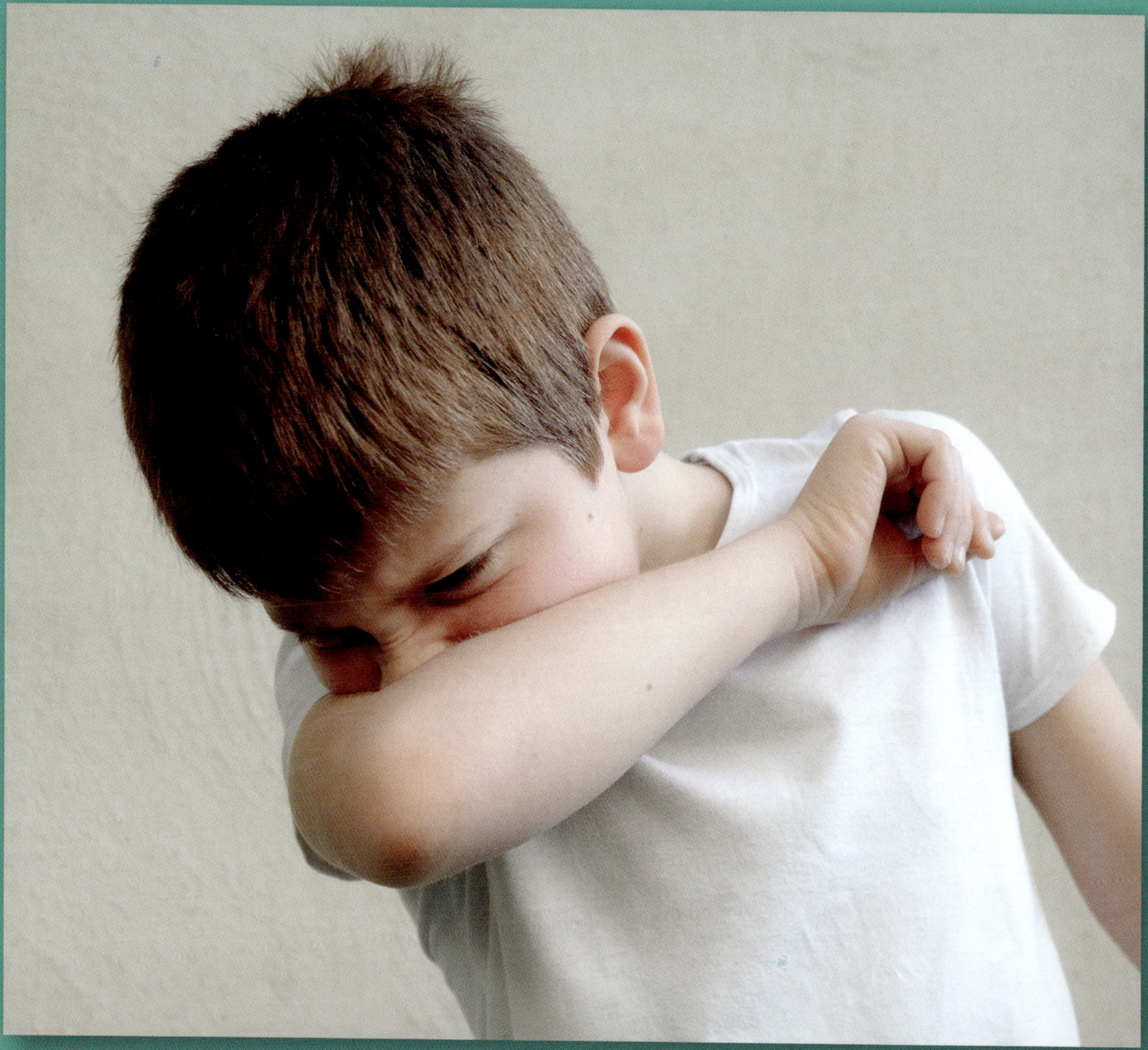

Cough into the bend of your arm, or inner elbow, to help prevent germs from spreading.

Healthy Habits

Did you know that some people have the coronavirus for up to 14 days before they know they're sick? Others don't have any **symptoms** at all, so they never even know they're infected! That means people can be **contagious** for weeks without ever knowing it. This is why it's important for *everyone* to practice healthy habits.

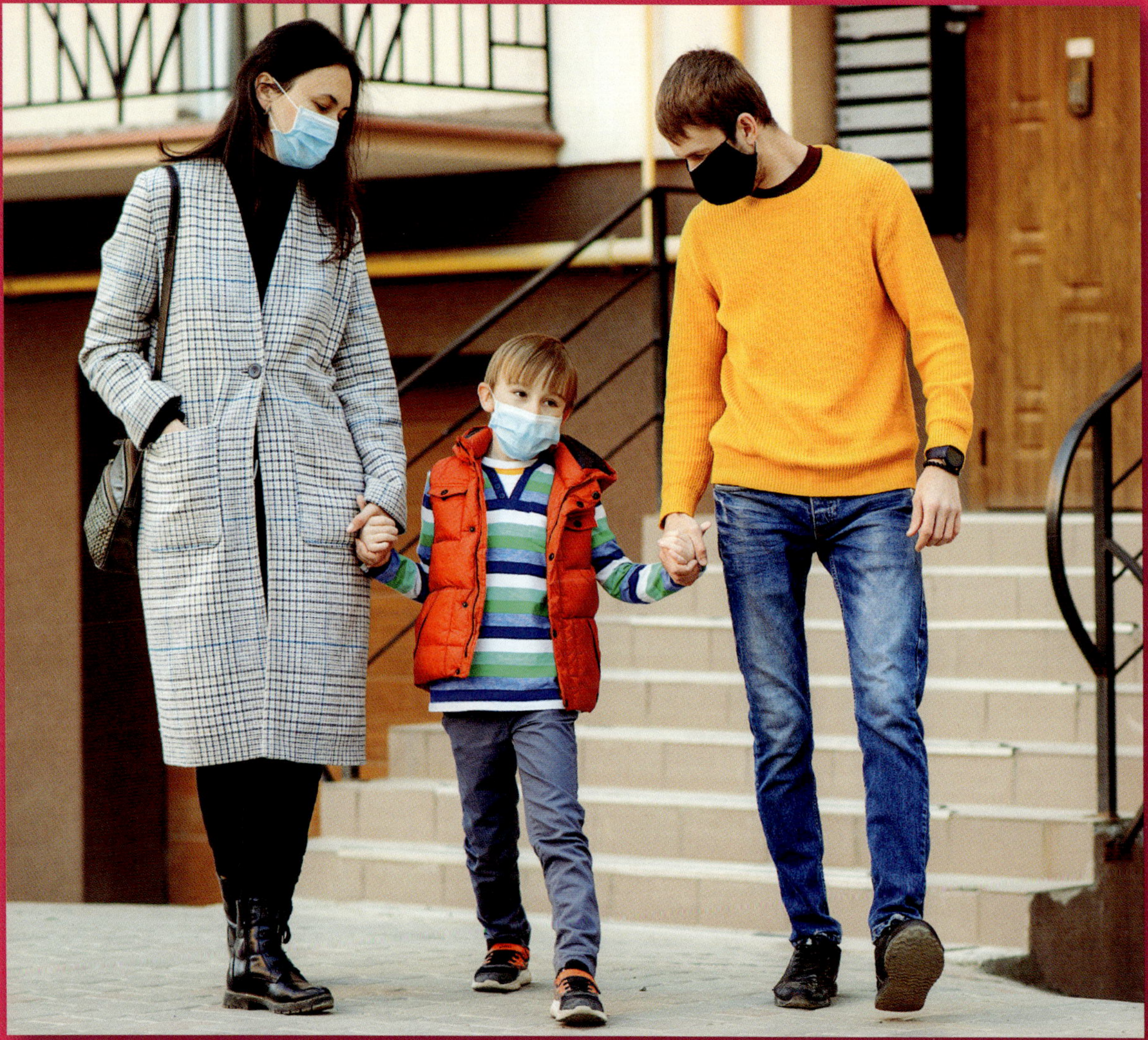

Be sure to wash or replace your mask often.

Although it's always safest to stay home during a pandemic, sometimes that's not an option. When you have to go out, practice social distancing and wear a cloth mask. Masks are especially important if you have to go someplace, like a store, where there are other people. Be sure to use hand sanitizer frequently while you're out. Then, when you get home, wash with soap and water.

Look!

If you see other people approaching while going on a walk, safely cross to the other side of the road. That way, you will stay at least 6 feet (2 meters) away.

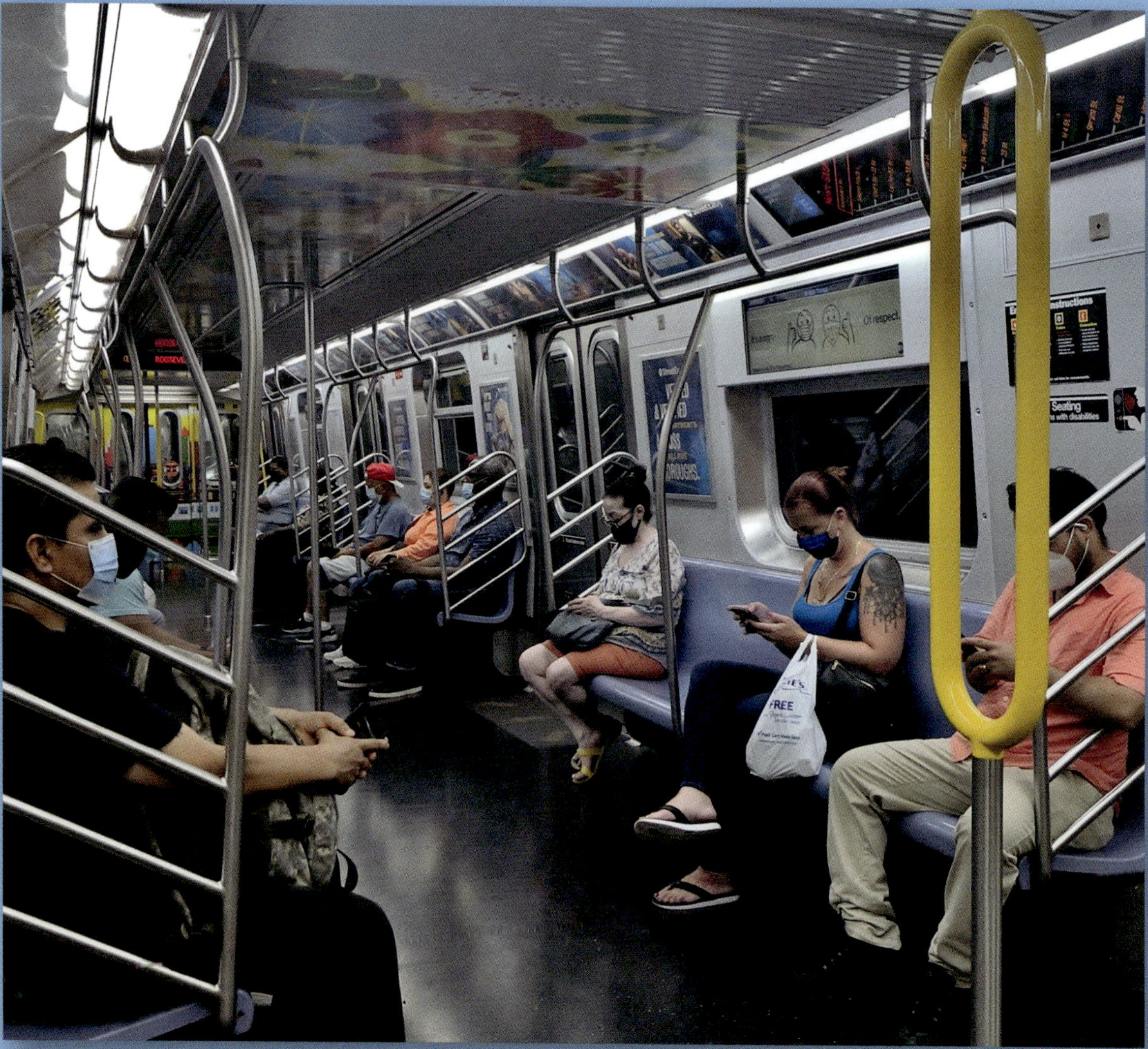

If you must ride the subway or a bus, put as much room between you and others as possible.

There is still so much we don't know about the new coronavirus. Some researchers believe that virus droplets can float in the air for several hours. Others have found that the virus can survive for up to 7 days on certain surfaces, like metal doorknobs and silverware. Are items being delivered to your home? You can be certain that it's safe to bring them inside once you've wiped them down with a damp, soapy cloth. After everything has been put away, help clean the counters with **disinfectant** and wash your hands.

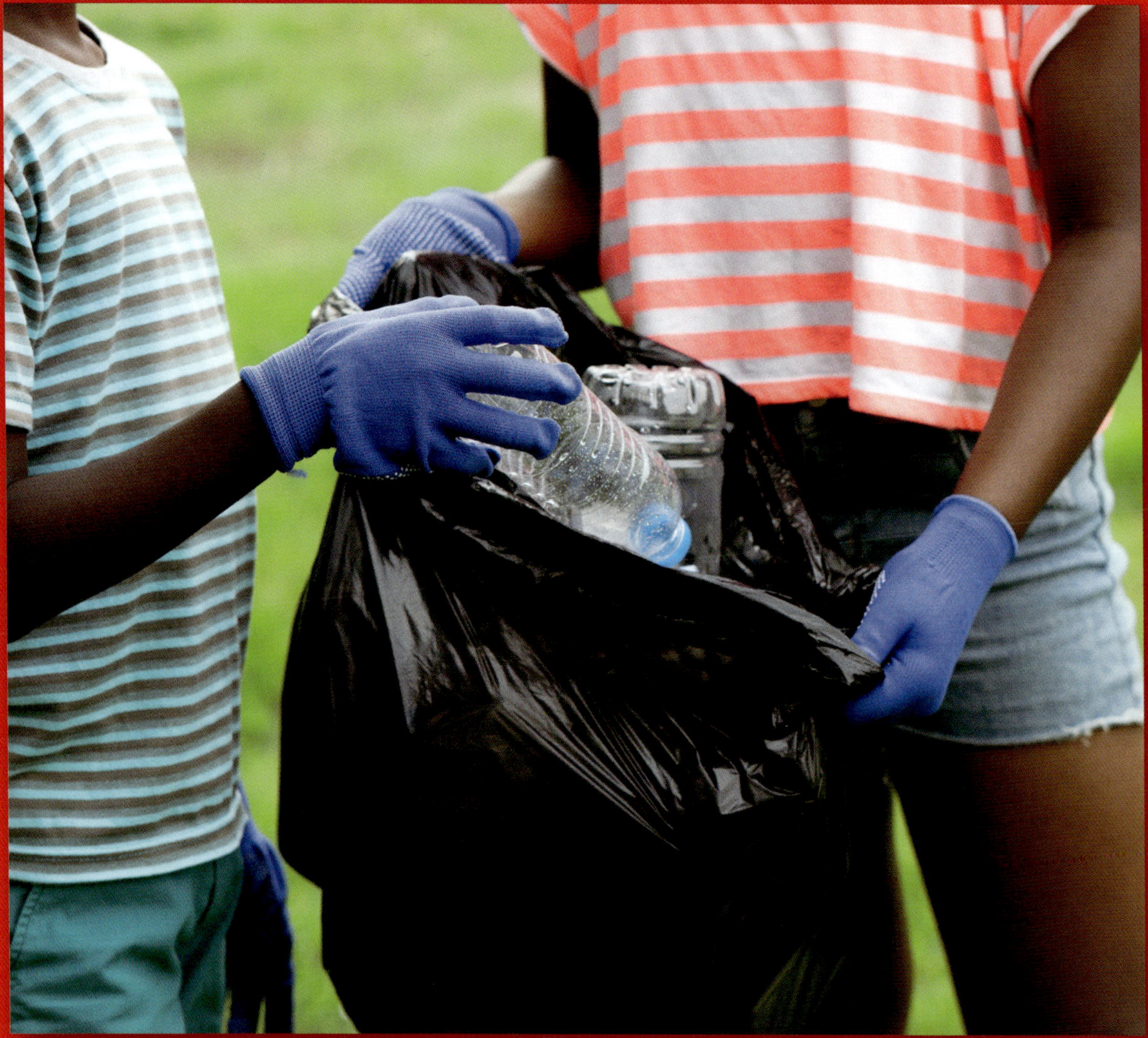

To help keep your neighborhood clean, pick up trash wearing gloves. Always wash your hands for 20 seconds when you're done!

Staying healthy also means taking care of your mind and your heart. Be sure to name your feelings. Share them with grown-ups, write them down in a journal, and give yourself permission to be sad sometimes. And always remember, you're not alone!

Create!

When you do art or make music, happy chemicals are released in your brain. During quarantine, try to find a way to be creative every day. Do what you love!

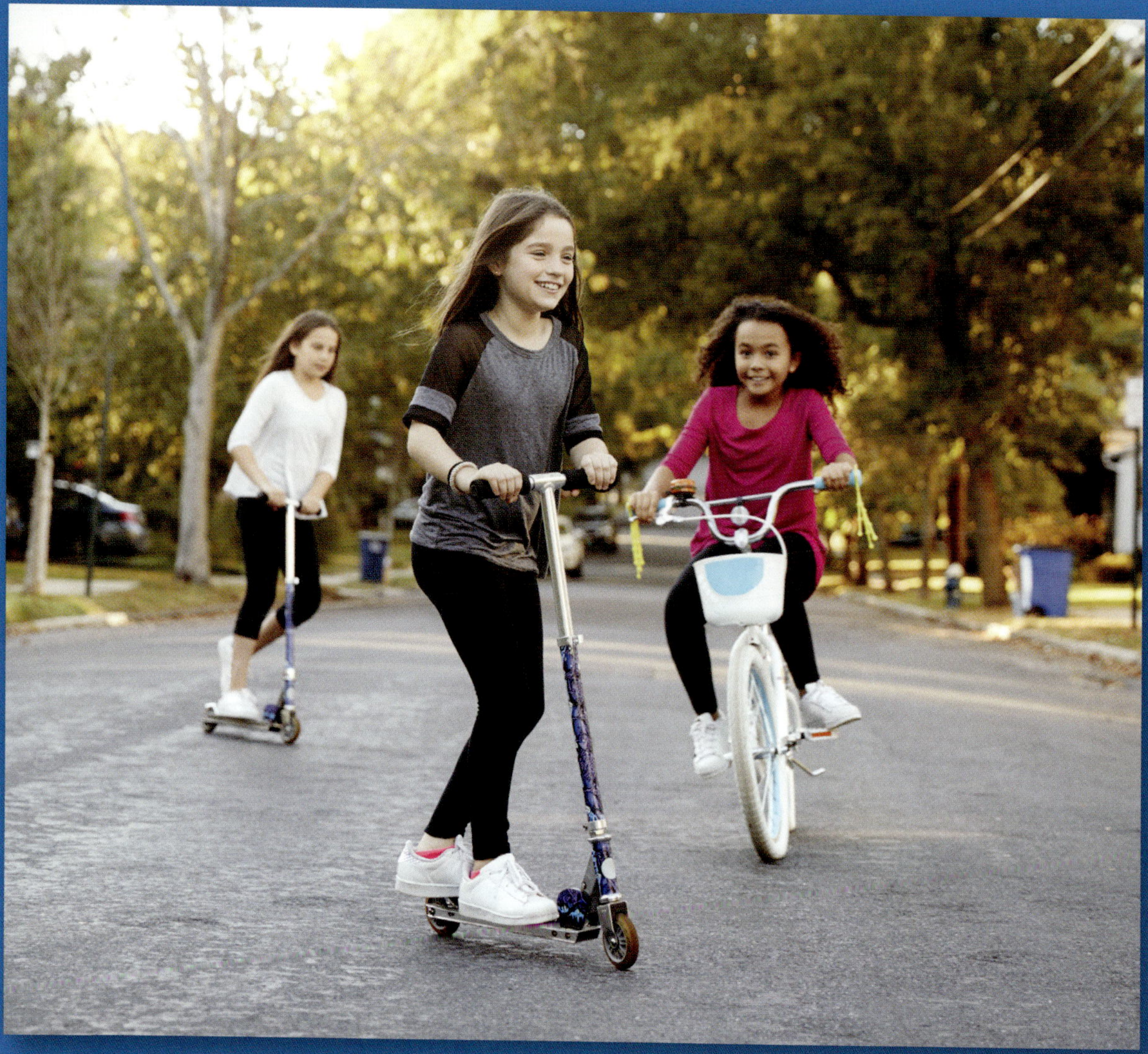

Try to stay at least 6 feet (2 m) away from friends when you're outside.

Healthy with Friends

Although it's not safe to have playdates indoors during a pandemic, you can still see friends and family members from a distance. Take walks or bike rides on opposite sides of the street. Socially distanced hikes or chats and visits using technology are also wonderful ways to have healthy visits. If you play games during one of these visits, just make sure you're not touching the same objects. Sadly, games like tag and frisbee will have to wait.

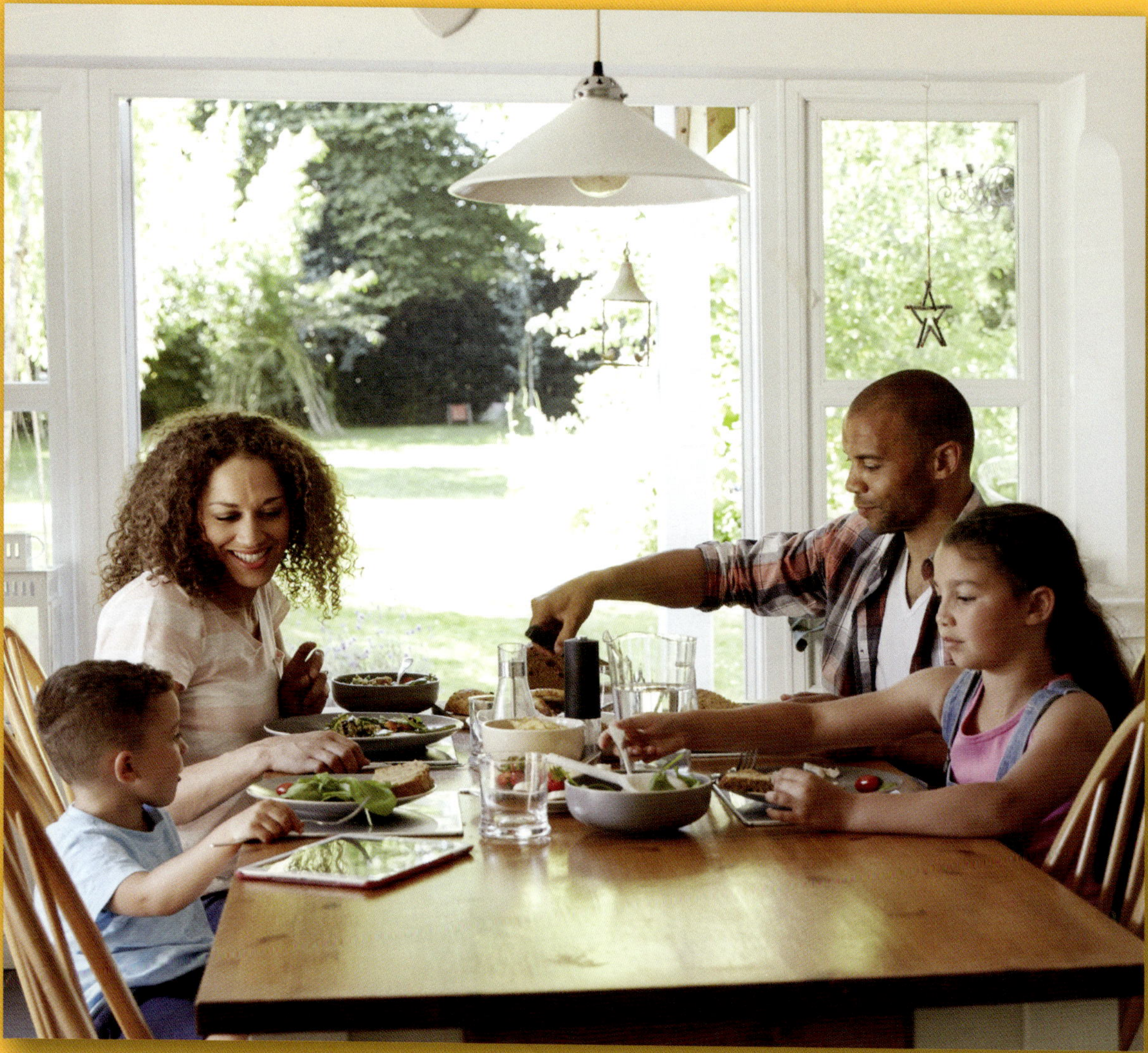

Families who eat meals together stay healthy and happy together.

Is it safe to pet someone else's dog right now? The short answer is no. Unfortunately, there is still so much to learn about this virus, including whether it can be passed to people from animals' fur. The best way to make sure everyone stays healthy is to wave or maybe blow a kiss from a safe distance away. Remember, pandemics don't last forever. The better we are about taking steps to stay healthy, the sooner we'll be free to pet all the dogs we want to again!

Think!

Can you think of a game you can play from a safe distance?

GLOSSARY

contagious (kuhn-TAY-juhs) able to be spread from one person to another, through direct or indirect contact

coronavirus (kuh-ROH-nuh-vye-ruhs) a family of viruses that cause a variety of illnesses in people and other mammals

disinfectant (dis-in-FEK-tuhnt) a cleaning product that can be used on surfaces to kill viruses

hygiene (HYE-jeen) the practice of keeping yourself and your environment clean to maintain good health

pandemic (pan-DEM-ik) an outbreak of a disease that affects a large part of the population

quarantined (KWOR-uhn-teend) isolated from others

social distancing (SOH-shuhl DIS-tuhns-ing) the act of staying at least 6 feet (2 meters) away from others

symptoms (SIMP-tuhmz) signs of an illness

FIND OUT MORE

WEBSITES

Action for Healthy Kids—COVID-19 and At-Home Resources
https://www.actionforhealthykids.org/covid-19-and-at-home-resources

CDC—What You Should Know About COVID-19 to Protect Yourself and Others
https://www.cdc.gov/coronavirus/2019-ncov/downloads/2019-ncov-factsheet.pdf

Food & Fun After School—Planning for the Week
http://foodandfun.org/?p=learn/parents/info&subject=Planning+for+the+Week

The Foundation for Global Community Health—Brain Breaks
https://brain-breaks.com

GoNoodle—Move and Learn at Home with Good Energy Summer
https://www.gonoodle.com/good-energy-at-home-kids-games-and-videos

Sciencing—How to Make a Simple 1-Minute Timer
https://sciencing.com/make-simple-minute-timer-5026941.html

INDEX

ABOUT THE AUTHOR

Shannon Stocker writes picture books, books for young readers, and *Chicken Soup* stories. She and her family try to stay healthy by wearing homemade cotton masks if they have to go out. Shannon lives in Louisville, Kentucky, with Greg, Cassidy, Tye, and far too many critters.